VET TOPICS

HOW TO HANDLE AN AFRICAN SWINE FEVER CRISIS

José Manuel Sánchez-Vicaíno Rodríguez
Cristina Jurado Díaz
Estefanía Cadenas Fernández

SERVET

Plaza Antonio Beltrán Martínez nº 1, planta 8 - letra I
(Centro empresarial El Trovador)
50002 Zaragoza - Spain

First printing: november 2019

This work is a translation of the book:
¿Cómo gestionar una crisis sanitaria de peste porcina africana?

Translation:
Owen Howard

ISBN: 978-84-18020-01-8
DL: Z 1862-2019

Design, layout and printing:
Servet editorial - Grupo Asís Biomedia, SL
www.grupoasis.com
info@grupoasis.com

Servet is the publishing house of Grupo Asís

Warning:

Veterinary science is constantly evolving, as are pharmacology and the other sciences. Inevitably, it is therefore the responsibility of the veterinary surgeon to determine and verify the dosage, the method of administration, the duration of treatment and any possible contraindications to the treatments given to each individual patient, based on his or her professional experience. Neither the publisher nor the author can be held liable for any damage or harm caused to people, animals or properties resulting from the correct or incorrect application of the information contained in this book.

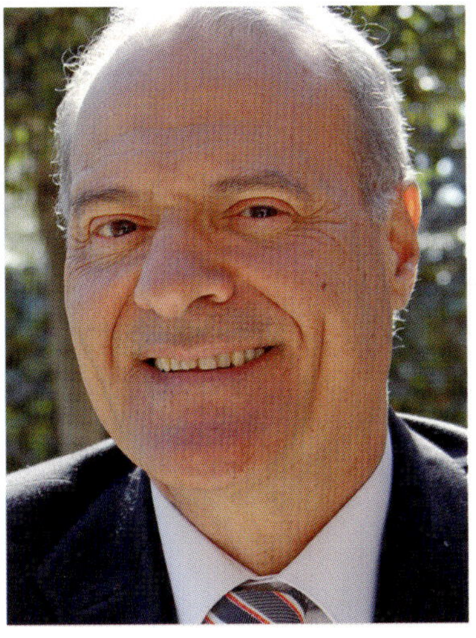

THE AUTHORS

José Manuel Sánchez-Vicaíno Rodríguez

Prof. Sánchez-Vizcaíno is professor of animal health at the Complutense University of Madrid (UCM), where he lectures and conducts research on infectious diseases in the Department of Animal Health of the Faculty of Veterinary Medicine. He is the director of the OIE reference laboratory for African swine fever. In 2013 he was nominated George Poppensiek visiting professor on global animal health at Cornell University, NY, USA. In September 2018 he was appointed adjunct professor of the Veterinary Population Medicine Department of the University of Minnesota.

Professor Sanchez-Vizcaíno's research has had a marked impact on the control and eradication of several animal diseases, including African swine fever, African horse sickness, and classical swine fever. His scientific contributions include new, fast, and sensitive diagnostic tests and reagents, as well as new epidemiological models and control strategies.

He has published over 200 articles in high-impact journals and has directed 27 PhD theses. In 2009 he was awarded the Merit Medal from the World Organisation for Animal Health in recognition of his outstanding services to veterinary science.

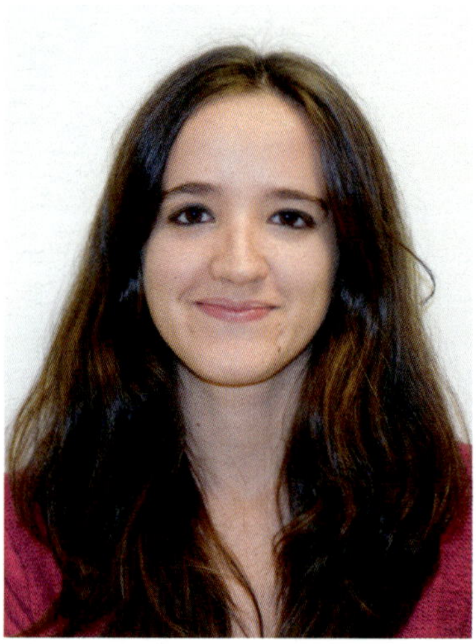

Cristina Jurado Díaz

Cristina Jurado Díaz received her degree in veterinary science from the Complutense University of Madrid (UCM), Spain (2014). During her senior year she worked as an intern developing new diagnostic techniques for African swine fever (ASF) using noninvasively acquired samples such as oral fluids. She subsequently joined the team of Prof. Sánchez-Vizcaíno at the OIE reference laboratory for ASF and VISAVET Health Surveillance Centre. In 2014 she began her PhD, which focused on the development of new epidemiological and diagnostic tools for the control and eradication of ASF in currently affected European territories. In the course of her studies she has acquired expertise on ASF in a research laboratory context, where she has learned how to perform diagnostic techniques and work in biosafety level 3 (BSL3) containment conditions. She has also gained experience in the epidemiology of ASF and the use of different tools (e.g. clustering techniques, time series studies, regression studies) to understand epidemiological scenarios. Since joining the team at UCM she has collaborated on several international and national projects, including ASFRISK, ASFORCE, and OIE twinning projects, and has published several scientific papers.

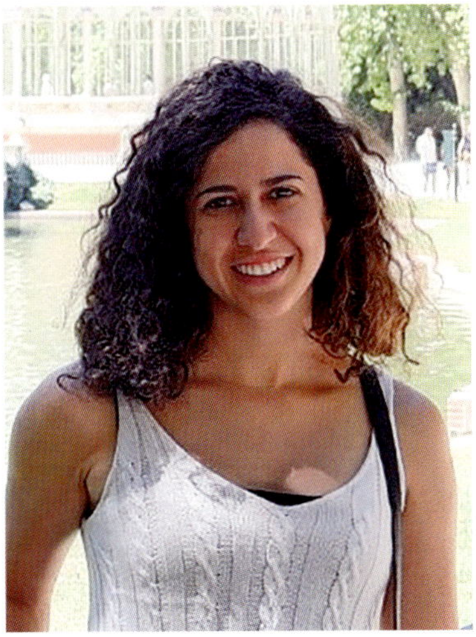

Estefanía Cadenas Fernández

Estefanía Cadenas Fernández holds a degree in veterinary science from the UCM (2017). Her interest in the health of wildlife and their interactions and impact on livestock led her in 2017 to pursue a master's degree in basic and applied research in hunting resources at the Spanish National Wildlife Research Institute (IREC-UCLM), where she acquired a basic knowledge of ecological, epidemiological, and statistical research tools. Upon completing her master's degree she joined Prof. Sánchez-Vizcaíno's team at the OIE Reference Laboratory for ASF and VISAVET Health Surveillance Centre. She was awarded a competitive PhD fellowship for the Training of Future Scholars (FPU) from the Spanish Ministry of Education, Culture and Sports. Her ongoing PhD studies focus on the development of new techniques for monitoring and controlling the spread of ASF between wild boar and domestic pigs. Since joining the team at UCM she has acquired expertise in laboratory research of ASF, including diagnostic techniques and working in BSL3 containment conditions, and in the evaluation of wildlife–livestock interactions in the context of ASF transmission.

PREFACE

The aim of this publication is to increase awareness and preparation for outbreaks of African swine fever (ASF). ASF is a haemorrhagic viral disease of domestic and wild Suidae and is deemed a notifiable disease by the World Organisation for Animal Health (OIE). Acute forms of ASF are characterised by high mortality rates (95–100 %) in the early stages of outbreaks in disease-free areas. Given the absence of any effective vaccine or treatment, ASF control strategies involve implementing strict sanitary measures, including slaughter of clinically affected animals and susceptible animals with which they have been in contact. Sanitary measures are accompanied by trade restrictions of varying scope that can lead to significant economic losses. Since its introduction into Georgia in 2007, ASF virus (ASFV) has spread to several European and Asian countries, affecting domestic pigs and wild boar alike.

The unprecedented spread of this disease through Eurasia, its devastating economic consequences in affected countries, and the high risk of outbreaks in neighbouring regions make ASF one of the greatest threats to the global swine industry. This book describes the key features of ASF including the characteristics of its causative agent (ASFV), its various routes of transmission, and the broad spectrum of clinical presentations, which include both acute and subclinical forms. In addition, it provides detailed information on the current distribution of the disease, the different epidemiological situations around the world, and regional differences in the most affected host species. Finally, the book discusses currently available tools for field detection and laboratory diagnosis of ASF, the importance of early detection, and recommended preventive and control measures. The contents will be useful to a broad range of readers with interest in the global pig industry, which faces a grave threat in the form of this transboundary disease.

TABLE OF CONTENTS

OVERVIEW OF AFRICAN SWINE FEVER

African swine fever (ASF) is considered one of the most dangerous diseases for the swine industry, owing to its socioeconomic consequences and its health impact. Animals infected with the ASF virus can present with internal and external haemorrhagic lesions, accompanied by fever that typically leads to anorexia, lethargy, and prostration. The economic consequences depend mainly on the commercial restrictions applied after notification of an outbreak or case of ASF, as well as on the sanitary measures established to eradicate foci on farms. ASF is deemed a notifiable disease by the World Organisation for Animal Health (OIE).

ASF is endemic in 28 countries on the African continent, and in the last decade has spread across much of Europe and reached Asia. Since its appearance in Georgia in 2007 it has spread through Eastern Europe via Armenia, Azerbaijan, Russia, Ukraine, and Belarus. The disease has been reported in 12 European countries since 2014, including Estonia, Latvia, Lithuania, Poland, Moldova, Romania, Bulgaria, Hungary, Belgium, the Czech Republic, Serbia, and Slovakia. Moreover, since 2018 ASF has spread to Asia, entering via China and reaching Mongolia, Vietnam, Cambodia, North Korea, Laos, and Myanmar in 2019.

According to official OIE notifications, both domestic pigs and wild boar have been affected, albeit in different proportions depending on the territory affected. Populations of wild boar, which are overly abundant, are severely affected by this disease. Indeed, wild boar are the primary host of ASF in the EU. It is therefore essential to establish efficient prevention and control measures that can reduce the incidence of ASF in affected territories. By contrast, outbreaks reported in Eastern Europe and Asia have almost exclusively occurred on domestic pig farms. Research should also seek to develop a safe and effective vaccine that will serve as a tool to curb this situation.

ASF VIRUS

ASF is a viral disease caused by the ASF virus (ASFV) that affects domestic and wild Suidae regardless of age and sex. ASFV is a large, complex, highly resistant double-stranded DNA virus. Owing to its complexity, its structure and the role of certain segments of its genome remain poorly understood.

ASFV exhibits great genetic variability: to date 24 different genotypes have been described. It should be noted that no link has been established between genotype and the virulence or evolution of viral isolates/strains. The virus also displays marked antigenic variability, and possesses a large number of viral proteins, some of which are highly immunogenic. However, antibodies synthesised by infected animals are unable to completely neutralise the virus.

Antibody synthesis begins between 7 and 12 days postinfection. These antibodies can persist for months or even years. Gradual changes in the response of infected animals have been observed over time in affected regions in Europe.

Characteristics of ASFV

- Large and highly complex.
- Great genetic and antigenic variability.
- Twenty-four distinct genotypes, with no link between genotype and virulence.
- Highly resistant in the environment.
- Variable clinical forms, ranging from acute and subacute to inapparent.
- Wide variety of specific and sensitive diagnostic techniques.
- No antibodies can completely neutralise the infection.
- No safe and effective treatment or vaccine exists.
- ASF is not a zoonotic disease.

Initially, infected animals in previously unexposed areas developed early viraemia. Subsequent sudden death prevented the development of antibodies against the virus. As the isolates circulated among susceptible populations an increase in the number of animals positive for anti-ASFV antibodies was observed. Viraemia was intermittent, and some animals even tested negative for the presence of virus in blood. Furthermore, clinical forms varied considerably, ranging from acute and subacute to inapparent, and survival rates increased.

DIAGNOSIS AND TREATMENT

Currently there is no commercial treatment or vaccine for ASF. The presence of antibodies against ASFV is always indicative of infection. Nowadays there are several techniques available that enable reliable diagnosis of ASF, and a wide variety of diagnostic techniques for the detection of the virus itself (e.g. real-time and conventional PCR) and of antibodies against the virus (e.g. enzyme-linked immunosorbent assay [ELISA], indirect immunoperoxidase assay, and Western blot). It is essential to use both types of diagnostic technique (direct and indirect) in parallel in order to obtain an overview of the epidemiological situation.

Given the absence of any vaccine against ASFV, disease control and eradication are achieved through the implementation of strict sanitary and containment measures.

> The application of preventive measures is crucial to avoid new cases/outbreaks, especially on farms, where adequate biosecurity is essential to prevent the entry and spread of ASF.

The effectiveness of these measures is influenced by several factors, including the location of the farm, the type of farm (intensive, extensive, or semi-extensive), the movement of animals, and the management system used. It is essential that pig farm workers are informed about the risk of entry of this disease, as well as the mechanisms by which it is transmitted.

Finally, it should be noted that ASF does not affect humans, and therefore has a limited impact on public health.

TRANSMISSION MECHANISMS

ASF can be transmitted via direct or indirect contact between infected and susceptible animals (domestic pigs and/or wild boar). Therefore, contact with infectious fluids such as blood (in particular), secretions, and excretions (including faeces, especially when haemorrhagic) is a potential source of virus transmission. Transmission of the virus can also occur following consumption of contaminated meat or meat products (derived from infected animals). Historically, this has been one of the most common routes by which the virus has been introduced into countries. Examples include Portugal (1957, 1960) and Georgia (2007).

ASFV can also be transmitted by the bite of soft ticks of the genus *Ornithodoros*. ASFV is transmitted by ticks of the species *Ornithodoros erraticus* in Spain and Portugal, and in Africa by *Ornithodoros moubata*. To date, all studied species of the genus *Ornithodoros* appear to be capable of transmitting ASFV. In addition to *O. erraticus* and *O. moubata*, these include *Ornithodoros porcinus*, *Ornithodoros coriaceus*, *Ornithodoros turicata*, and *Ornithodoros savignyi*. Other *Ornithodoros* species have been identified in other territories including the United States and Latin America. However, a lack of knowledge regarding the precise geographic distribution of these vectors limits understanding of their role in affected areas such as Europe or Asia.

Academic research, including studies conducted in Sardinia and Germany, has sought to resolve these doubts by using ELISA techniques to detect pigs and wild boar bitten by these ticks and by capturing vectors using dry-ice traps. The results obtained indicate an apparent absence of these vectors in the areas studied.

The role of fomites

One of the characteristics that favour the transmission of ASFV is its high level of resistance in the environment. Consequently, fomites play an important role in ASFV transmission. The presence of contaminated vehicles, incorrect changing of clothes and/or footwear when entering farms, and the sharing of instruments between farms are just some of the critical parameters to control in order to prevent the entry and dissemination of ASF. Transmission of the virus through contact with stable flies (*Stomoxys calcitrans*) has also been described. These flies act as mechanical vectors (for periods of up to 12–24 hours). A recent study demonstrated the transmission of ASFV through the ingestion of flies, although this appears to be uncommon. Taken together these findings underscore the importance of taking precautions when carrying out necropsies on farms, implementing appropriate disinsection programmes, and using mosquito nets in the windows of facilities in which animals are housed.

DISEASE PRESENTATION

ASF is a haemorrhagic disease that does not cause pathognomonic lesions. Although some lesions can be very significant, the differential diagnosis should always include other diseases with similar clinical signs, including classical swine flu, erysipelas, and septicaemic diseases such as salmonellosis.

Hunting

The implementation of disease-control protocols during hunting activities has become increasingly important in recent years. Appropriate handling of carcasses and offal, vehicle cleaning and disinfection, and changing of clothing and footwear are crucial to ensure disease control, especially in cases of hunters who also work on pig farms.

> The clinical form varies depending on the virulence of the circulating isolate, the route of infection, and certain host-specific factors such as age and species.

In general the incubation period ranges from 3 to 19 weeks. The associated clinical signs consist of fever, lethargy, anorexia, weakness, erythema and, in extreme cases, haemorrhage. Internal lesions may affect various organs. Splenomegaly, haemorrhagic lymph nodes, and the presence of fluid in the pericardial, thoracic, and abdominal cavities are relatively common (Figs. 1–3). Isolates of moderate virulence predominantly cause acute and subacute clinical presentations. These cases are characterised by fluctuating fever peaks lasting 2–3 weeks and less severe clinical signs. Mortality rates can range from 30–70 %, and deaths usually occur around 20 days after infection.

ASFV isolates capable of inducing subclinical and inapparent infections have also been described. Affected animals show seroconversion and intermittent viraemia, and mortality rates are low. This clinical presentation has been observed in endemic scenarios, in which clinical signs can be very mild or even absent. Due to the potential role of these animals as carriers of disease, it is essential to establish a correct diagnosis that includes parallel detection of both the virus and antibodies.

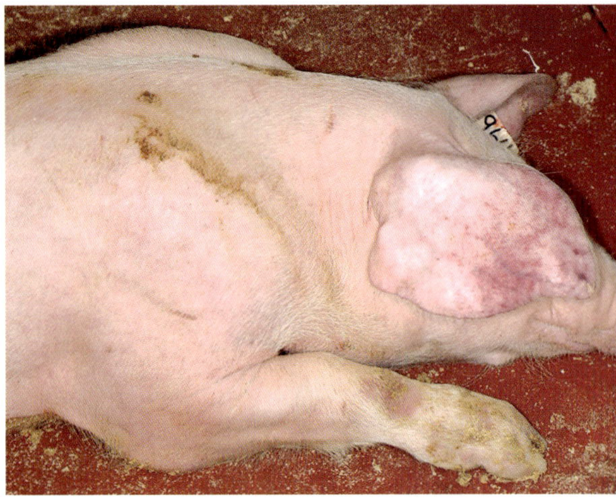

Figure 1. Redness and cyanosis around the ear margins in a domestic pig.

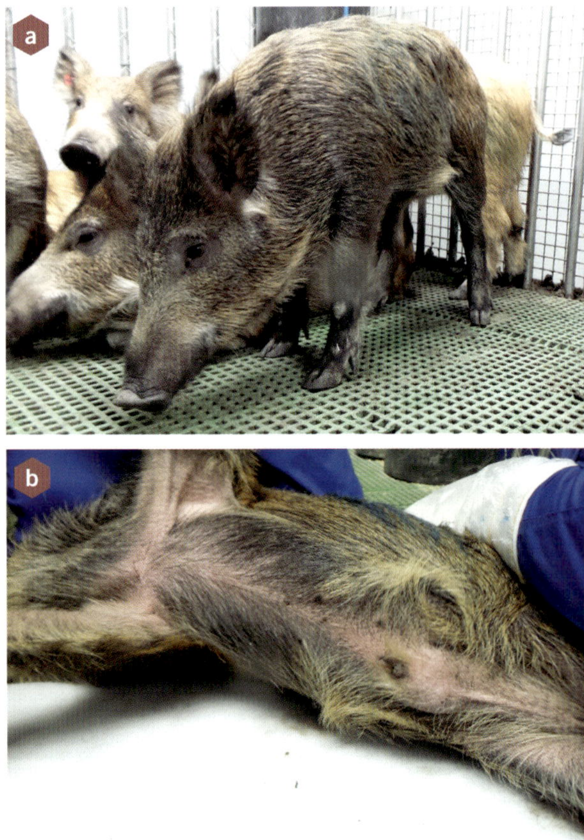

Figure 2. European wild boar in which (a) depression and (b) erythema on the ventral surface are evident.

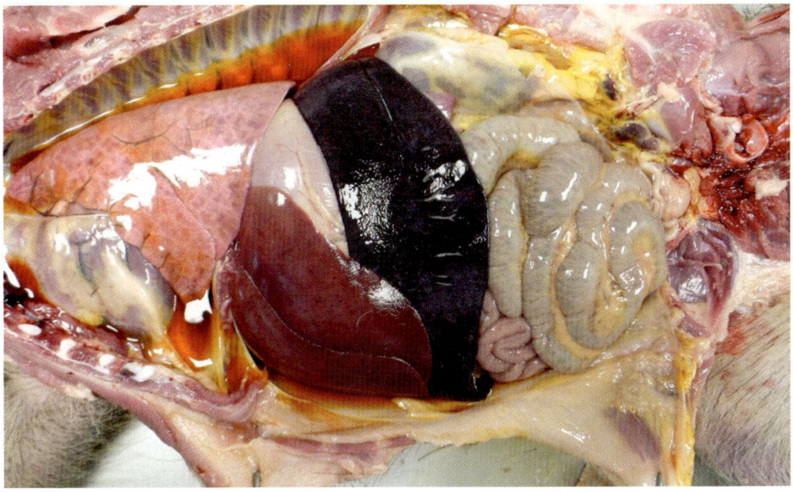

Figure 3. Presence of free fluid in the thoracic cavity, hypertrophied spleen crossing the abdominal surface, and presence of oedematous intestinal loops.

PREVENTION AND CONTROL

The implementation of preventive measures is crucial to prevent the entry and spread of infectious diseases. There is no single solution to prevent ASF entry into a given area. The success of preventive measures is directly influenced by factors such as the type of host (domestic pigs and/or wild boar), the presence of vectors, the existence of up-to-date contingency plans for the disease in question, financial resources, and the availability of personnel.

It is also essential to have up-to-date epidemiological information from neighbouring countries and those with which there are direct commercial relations.

Control measures

- Reduce or avoid, to the extent possible, the purchase of live animals or their products from risk areas.
- Strict precautions should be applied to the transport of animals, ensuring proper cleaning and disinfection of the vehicles used.
- Overabundance of wild boar should be controlled by reducing the population.
- Review contingency plans.
- Reinforce training of veterinary professionals to ensure correct recognition of the disease.
- Conduct awareness campaigns in order to reach the maximum number of segments within the pig industry.
- Review and update potential entry routes based on existing production systems.
- Continue and strengthen research efforts to develop a safe and effective vaccine against the virus.

Disease control in wild boar requires restoration of the population balance as well as rapid and safe removal of carcasses from the environment. Control of outbreaks on farms requires strict implementation of control and eradication measures, correct removal of carcasses, and cleaning and disinfection of facilities and vehicles.

This information allows authorities to make risk-based decisions and promote continuing education programmes targeting multiple levels, including professionals working in the pig industry, public and private veterinary practitioners, hunters, and the general public.

The effectiveness of control measures will depend on the diligence with which potential signs of ASF are monitored, the time taken to establish diagnosis, and the time elapsed before containment measures are implemented. Failures in disease control can result from certain cultural practices such as domestic animal slaughter, the sale of infected products, and taboos around wasting food in some cultures.

Vaccines are one of the most important tools for the control of infectious diseases. Unfortunately, no safe and effective commercial vaccine against ASFV is currently available. Great efforts are being made to develop a prototype vaccine capable of preventing the spread of this disease. At the Complutense University of Madrid, Spain, research is being conducted in collaboration with the Animal Health Research Centre of the National Institute for Agricultural and Food Research and Technology (CISA-INIA) to develop an effective oral vaccine for wild boar. Results obtained to date indicate protection values of approximately 92 %. These promising results offer hope of the development of yet another tool for use in the fight against ASF.

CURRENT EPIDEMIOLOGICAL SCENARIOS

Currently, African swine fever (ASF) is a cause of great concern within the swine industry and for veterinary authorities worldwide. It is widely distributed in three continents (Africa, Europe, and Asia), with varying epidemiological patterns depending on virus–vector–host interactions.

The study of these epidemiological patterns is of great importance for the development and implementation of prevention and control measures.

AFRICA

ASF is named after the African continent, where the first recorded case was detected in Kenya in 1921. Since then the disease has remained endemic in most sub-Saharan countries (Fig. 1).

In Africa, two distinct epidemiological cycles can be distinguished:

- A very complex epidemiological cycle is described in the southeast region of the African continent, characterised by the coexistence of wild Suidae, such as warthogs (*Phacochoerus aethiopicus*) and the red river hog (*Potamochoerus porcus*), soft ticks belonging to the *Ornithodoros moubata* complex, and domestic pigs. Wild Suidae are abundant in Southeast Africa and, unusually, are tolerant to ASF; they are capable of maintaining such low levels of the virus in blood that they do not develop the disease. They therefore serve as reservoirs and a permanent source of the virus. The ASF virus (ASFV) can replicate in ticks of the *O. moubata* complex. These act as vectors, transmitting the virus between wild Suidae and domestic pigs. All 24 of the ASFV genotypes described to date have been identified in this region.
- A second, less complex epidemiological cycle that exclusively involves domestic pigs is described in the central and western areas of the continent. Transmission occurs via contact between infected and susceptible animals and the consumption of contaminated pork products. In central Africa, specifically in Malawi, *Ornithodoros porcinus* has also been implicated in the transmission of ASFV in domestic pigs. To date, only one ASFV genotype (genotype I) has been identified in central and western Africa.

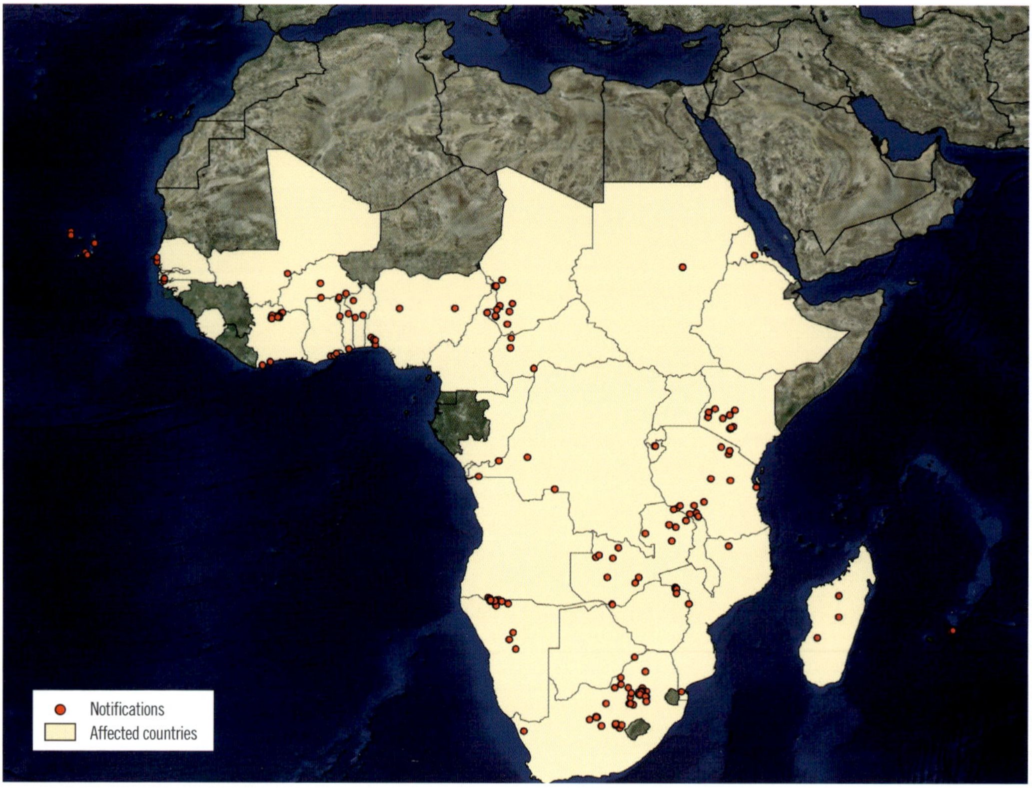

Figure 1. Map showing ASF notifications in Africa from 1994 to September 2019, highlighting the affected countries.

EUROPE

ASF has long been present in Europe. Its arrival through Portugal in 1957 led to the first recorded outbreak outside of the African continent, although this outbreak was quickly controlled. Three years later, in 1960, the disease again appeared in Portugal and spread throughout the country, subsequently affecting Spain. After more than 15 years of relative stability on the Iberian Peninsula, a large number of outbreaks occurred in previously ASF-free countries in Europe (France, Malta, Belgium, the Netherlands, and Italy, including the island of Sardinia) and the Americas (Dominican Republic, Haiti, Cuba, and Brazil). All the countries affected at that time managed to eradicate the disease during the 1990s, except for the island of Sardinia, where ASF has been present since 1978.

In 2007 ASF re-entered Europe, this time through Georgia, from where the disease spread northwards reaching Armenia, Azerbaijan, and Russia that same year. From Russia, ASF spread to Ukraine (2012), Belarus (2013), Estonia (2014), Latvia (2014), Lithuania (2014), and Poland (2014). Between 2016 and 2019, eight other countries notified the OIE of the presence of ASF (Fig. 2), specifically Moldova (2016), Romania (2017), the Czech Republic (2017), Hungary (2018), Bulgaria (2018), Belgium (2018), Slovakia (2019), and Serbia (2019). Currently, there is a very high risk of ASF outbreak in neighbouring countries, including France, Germany, and Spain. Given that

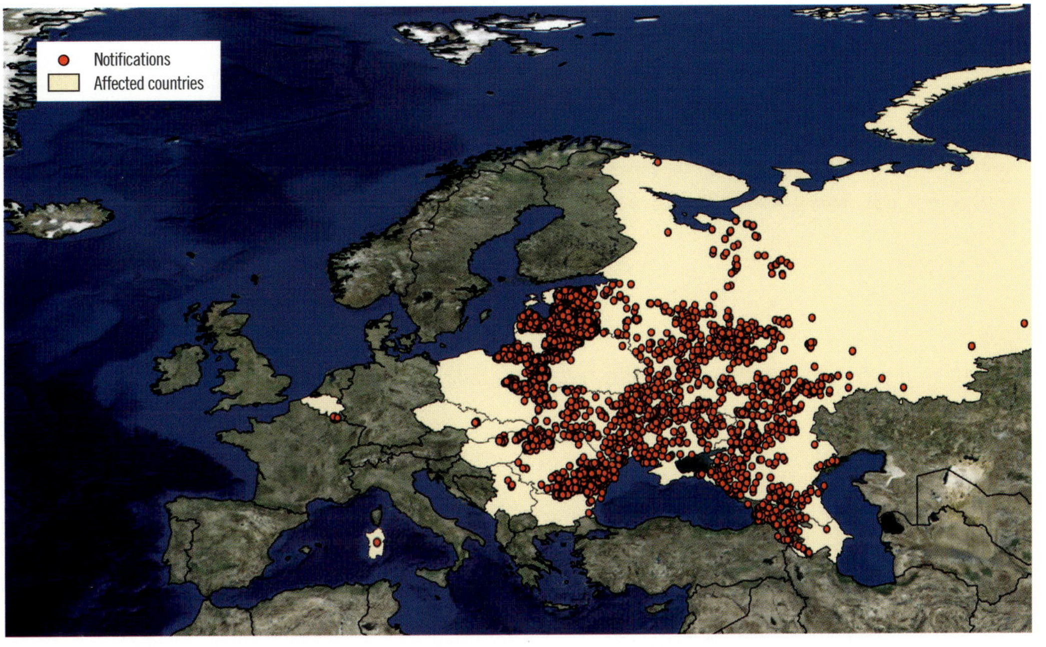

Figure 2. ASF notifications to the OIE by European countries between January 2007 and September 2019.

Germany and Spain are Europe's largest pig producers, ASF outbreaks in these countries could lead to huge economic losses.

In Europe, both domestic pigs and wild boar have been affected. Unlike wild Suidae in Africa, wild boar in Europe are susceptible to ASF, and develop a clinical presentation very similar to that observed in domestic pigs. The key role played by wild boar in ASF transmission in Europe is a result of their overabundance in this area. This in turn significantly influences several determinants of disease transmissibility, including the rate of contact between individuals. The ASF outbreaks in Spain and Portugal were characterised by an epidemiological cycle involving ticks of the species *O. erraticus*. However, the presence of these ticks in other affected countries has not been demonstrated, and they appear not to be involved in current epidemic scenarios. Transmission of the virus occurs through direct and indirect contact between susceptible and infected animals (domestic pigs and/or wild boar), consumption by animals of contaminated meat and meat products, and contact with vehicles and other fomites contaminated with ASFV.

Within the European continent, two different epidemiological patterns are observed depending on the type of host predominantly affected. On the one hand, in affected countries within the European Union (with the exception of Romania, Bulgaria, and Slovakia) more than 90 % of reported cases have been attributed to wild boar infected with ASFV, with the remaining cases corresponding to sporadic outbreaks on domestic pig farms. However, in Eastern Europe, including Russia, Ukraine, Belarus, Moldova, and Romania, ASF predominantly affects domestic pig farms, and to a lesser extent wild boar (Fig. 3). One explanation for these distinct epidemiological patterns within Europe is the type of production system found in each region. European countries in which domestic pigs are mainly affected tend to have larger numbers of family or backyard farms.

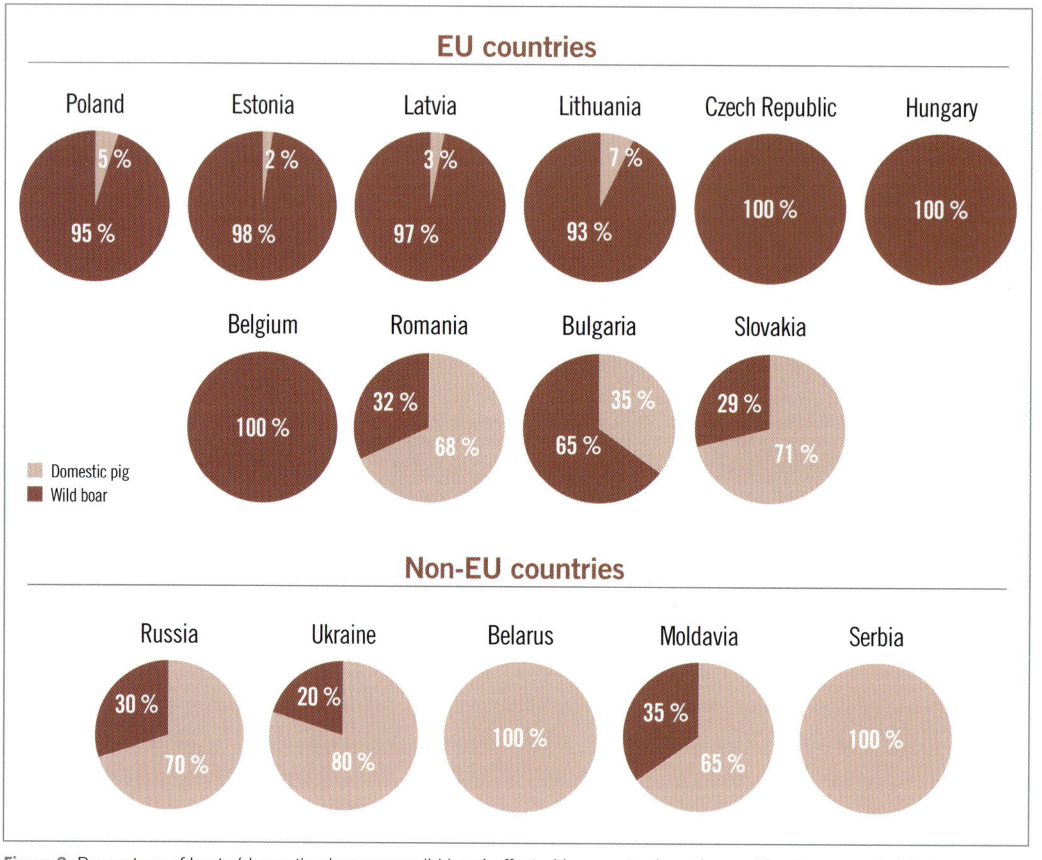

Figure 3. Percentage of hosts (domestic pigs versus wild boar) affected by country, based on notifications recorded between January 2007 and February 2019.

This type of production system usually has poor biosecurity and is usually found in areas in which wild boar live, increasing the risk of virus transmission. Moreover, pigs on these types of farms are sometimes fed with food waste, an activity that has historically been one of the main routes of ASFV transmission and is currently prohibited in the EU.

ASIA

The reintroduction of ASF to the European continent in 2007 has resulted in its spread through several European countries and, for the first time, to Asia. The first reported ASF outbreak in Asia occurred in China in early August 2018, on a domestic pig farm in the city of Shenyang. Epidemiological enquiries identified the importation of infected piglets and feeding of animals with contaminated food debris as possible sources of infection. The world's leading pig producer is China, which has over 400 million pigs (half of the world's pig population).

The spread of ASF through China has been considerably faster than other reported

The situation in Sardinia

The island of Sardinia is the region outside of Africa in which ASF has persisted the longest. Of the studied factors that account for the endemic status of ASF for more than 40 years on the island, the most significant is the traditional practice of raising free-range domestic pigs (i.e. pigs raised in extensive conditions with no veterinary controls), known in Sardinia as *brados*. The epidemiological cycle of ASF in Sardinia thus involves registered domestic pigs, *brados*, and wild boar. Fortunately, a role of soft ticks of the species *O. erraticus* in this cycle has been ruled out. However, *brados* act as a link between the populations of registered domestic pigs and wild boar, as evidenced by the high level of interaction between wild boar and these free-range domestic pigs revealed by camera trap studies (Fig. 4). This situation has greatly facilitated the spread and persistence of the virus among susceptible hosts on the island. Domestic pig farms and wild boar account for similar proportions of disease notifications. A recently published study on the health status of *brados* showed a much higher viral and serological prevalence in these animals than in registered domestic pigs and wild boar. Multiple epidemiological studies carried out in the area confirmed the role of free-range pigs in maintaining the endemic status of ASF in Sardinia. This led to prohibition of this practice in 2012, and a subsequent campaign to eliminate these animals from the island. The progressive reduction of this population has coincided with a marked decrease in the number of outbreaks/cases in both domestic pigs and wild boar, indicating that the eradication of ASF in Sardinia appears to be a matter of time.

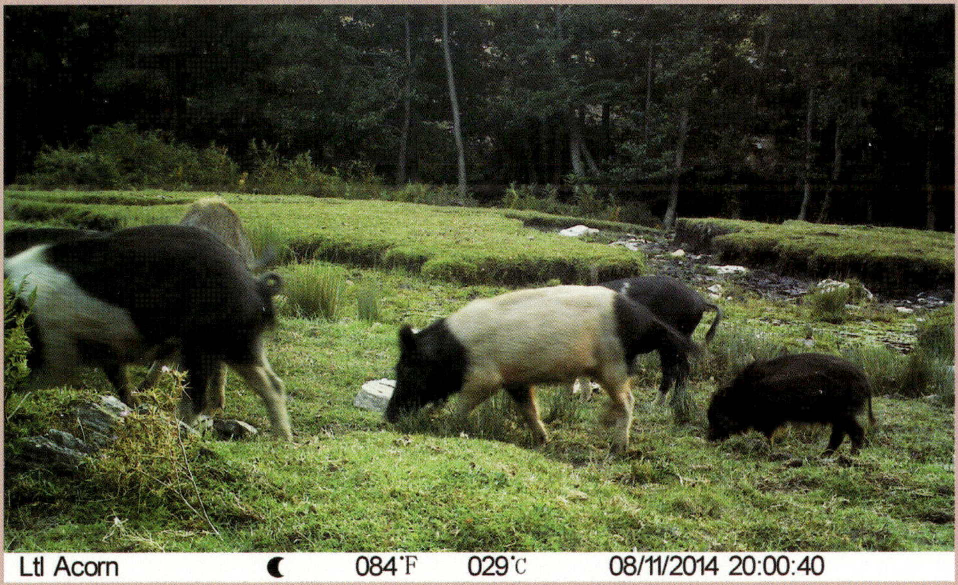

Figure 4. Interaction between free-range pigs and wild boar on the island of Sardinia, as captured by camera trap.

epidemics: in just 1 year more than 150 outbreaks occurred in 32 different provinces, with devastating effects on the country's economy (Fig. 5). This rapid spread of ASF has also been observed elsewhere in Asia: in 2019 eight more countries reported the presence of ASF (Mongolia, Vietnam, Cambodia, Hong Kong, North Korea, Laos, Myanmar, and the Philippines). Of these, Vietnam has been the most severely affected, with more than 6,000 outbreaks in 62 different provinces, requiring the slaughter of over 4.5 million pigs.

One important aspect of the spread of ASF throughout the Asian continent is the high estimated density of wild boar in this region, which is even higher than that of the EU. This is of particular epidemiological relevance: as described in Europe, wild boar may play a crucial role in the endemic status and maintenance of ASF in Asia. To date, only three cases have been reported in wild boar: two in the Chinese province of Jilin and another on a wild boar farm of 222 animals in the province of Inner Mongolia.

Notifications of outbreaks separated by hundreds of kilometres suggest that the transport of infected animals has facilitated the rapid spread of ASF. Furthermore, products made from Chinese pork that has tested positive for ASFV by PCR have been found in passenger luggage

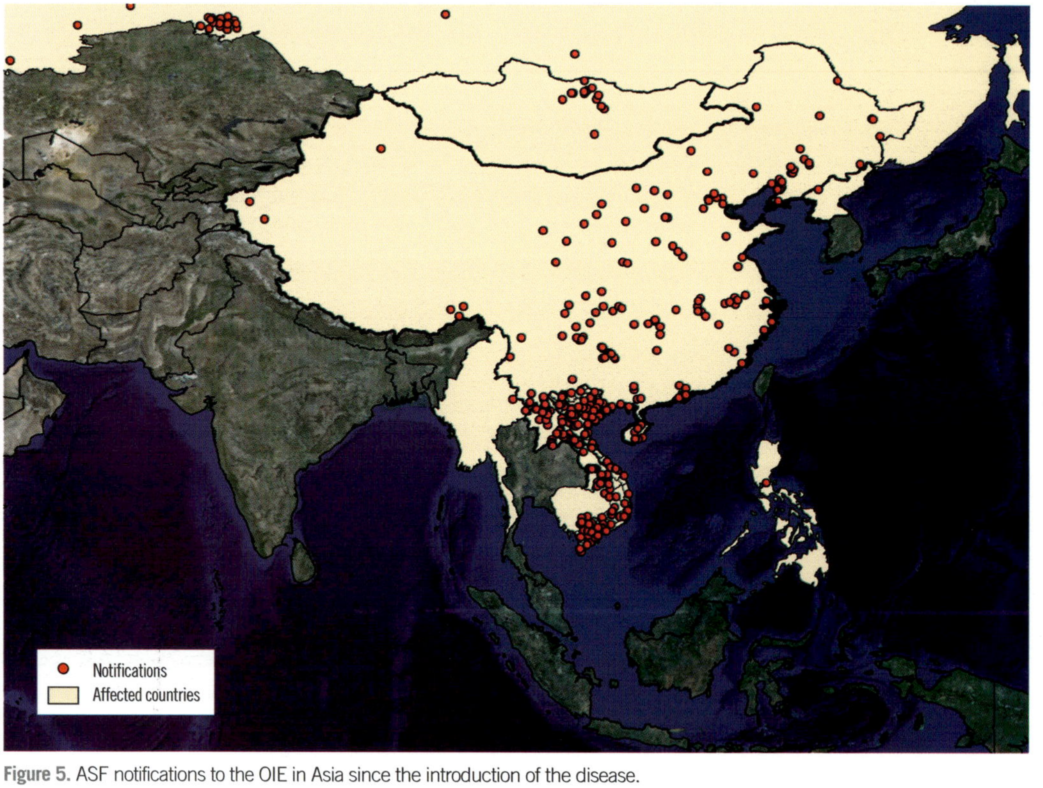

Figure 5. ASF notifications to the OIE in Asia since the introduction of the disease.

in airports in South Korea, Japan, Thailand, Taiwan, and Australia. Only Japan has compiled official data on the viability of the virus and the infective capacity of the confiscated products. This situation underscores a clear need to increase surveillance measures and preparation for ASF outbreaks.

FUTURE PERSPECTIVES

The information presented here leaves no doubt that ASF poses a serious threat, and constitutes one of the greatest dangers to animal health within the global swine industry. Affected countries have suffered huge economic losses due to the implementation of strict sanitary measures and the imposition of trade barriers. Moreover, in a large number of disease-free countries the risk of infection is very high. Because Asia and Europe account for more than 80 % of the global pig population, the control and eradication of ASF should be a priority for the pig industry worldwide. The current epidemic status of ASF will likely have important implications for the future of pig farming.

An important point to note is that human activity is the main source of ASFV transmission to new regions: the primary causes of virus introduction are feeding of pigs with food waste, contaminated vehicles, and poor biosecurity measures. ASF outbreaks are more frequent in countries in which family or backyard farms account for a large proportion of national pig production (e.g. Vietnam, Romania). A likely consequence of this phenomenon is that this type of production will give way to intensive systems.

Close attention should also be paid to the role that wild boar play in ASF transmission. Wild boar populations are susceptible to ASFV. However, veterinary control of wild populations is difficult. This fact, together with the high density of wild boar in Europe and Asia, sustains circulation of the virus among wild populations. Wild boar play a very important role in the maintenance and endemism of the disease, as evidenced by the epidemiological situation in certain EU countries.

Control of this disease is highly complex and requires a tremendous effort at all levels (field, administration, and research). One of the great challenges of ASF control and eradication is the absence of any treatment or commercial vaccine. For this reason, ASF research is focusing on the development of new control measures, including the development of a safe and effective ASFV vaccine. Historically, development of such a vaccine has been hampered by the great complexity of the virus, a lack of knowledge about virus–host interactions, the absence of a neutralising immune response, and technical difficulties including adaptation of the virus to a stable cell line.

Development of an effective and safe vaccine, together with establishment of adequate control and eradication plans, could provide the necessary means to curb the continued spread of the virus through Europe, Asia, and Africa, and to prevent its expansion into new territories.

EARLY DETECTION AND ACTION UPON SUSPICION OF ASF

African swine fever (ASF) is one of the diseases included in the list of notifiable diseases by the World Organisation for Animal Health (OIE). Notifications thus result in market restrictions at regional, national, and international levels. International restrictions have the greatest economic impact. Together with the results of risk analyses the current epidemiological situation, with over 50 countries in Africa, Europe, and Asia affected, confirms that ASF is one of the most dangerous diseases for pigs worldwide.

The following are the most likely routes by which ASFV can enter a disease-free country:

- Legal and illegal trade of live animals (domestic pigs and wild boar).
- Trade of meat and meat products.
- Contaminated modes of transport.
- Uncontrolled transport of contaminated products by tourists.
- Contaminated garbage and food debris from ships and airplanes (Fig. 1).
- Trade in semen and other pig products.
- Natural movement of wild animals (wild boar).

Why is ASF a notifiable disease?

The OIE has compiled a single list of notifiable diseases, each of which must meet the following criteria:

- The disease has a serious economic and health impact, the latter of which is related to its morbidity or mortality in domestic or wild animals.
- International propagation of the pathogen through live animals, their products, vectors, or fomites has been demonstrated.
- At least one country has demonstrated the effective absence of the disease in susceptible populations.
- Transmission to humans with serious consequences has been demonstrated.

ASF fulfils the first three criteria, but lacks zoonotic potential, limiting its impact on public health.

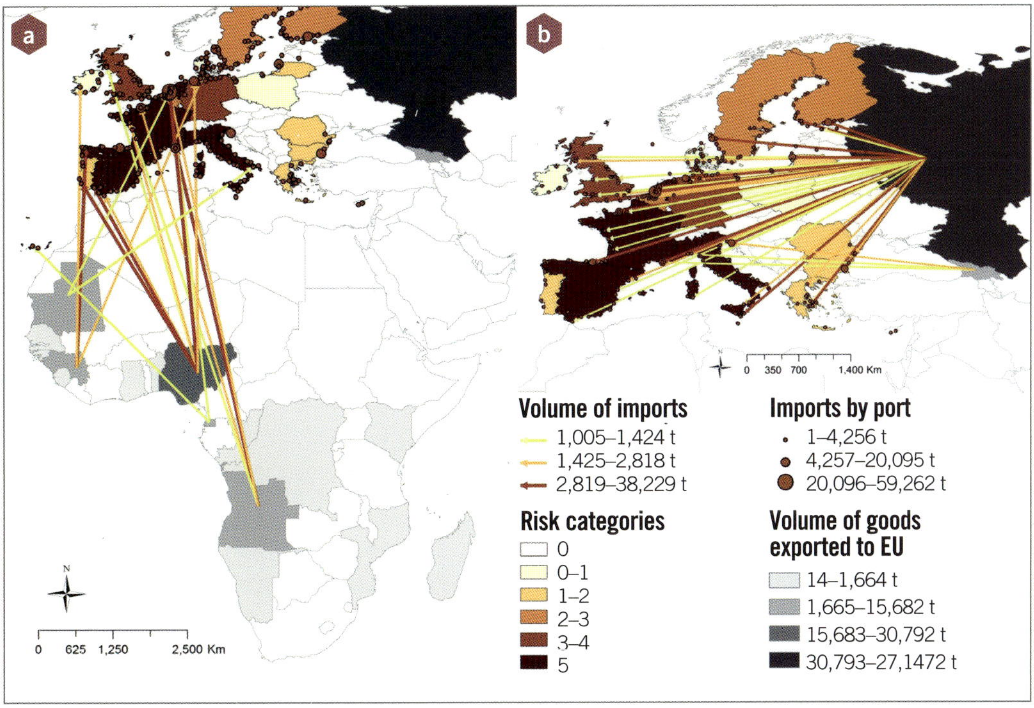

Figure 1. Relative risk of the introduction of the African swine fever virus (ASFV) into the European Union (EU) from food scraps on cargo ships. Image shows (a) the origin and destination of ships travelling from Africa and (b) European countries affected by ASF (Mur et al., 2012b).

- Biological vectors.
- Fomites.
- Release from laboratories that work with these pathogens.
- Bioterrorism.

HOW SHOULD WE PREPARE?

Suspicion and early detection in the field are crucial minimise or stop, to the extent possible, problems caused by the entry of new diseases, particularly in the case of ASF. The main factors that can improve and expedite the response to these types of diseases are continuous training and the dissemination of up-to-date epidemiological information to veterinary practitioners.

In any area, adequate prevention requires detailed information on existing hazards, as well as the level of risk associated with these threats. In short, for the purposes of prevention and preparation, risk analysis studies are very useful tools, and can help provide answers to the following questions: What is the most likely route of introduction into a specific territory? When is this most likely to occur? Where is it most likely to happen?

> Risk analysis is the systematic process of collecting and scientifically evaluating relevant information about a specific danger (in this case, a pathogen) in order to estimate the probability of its introduction, consequent disease, and the impact thereof.

Risk analyses are scientific studies that identify routes of introduction, periods during which pathogen entry is more likely, and areas most likely to be affected, and quantify the risk and consequences of exposure (Fig. 2). They are vital tools for establishing an effective, risk-based surveillance programme. Furthermore, risk analysis is the only scientific tool upon which we can rely to justify closing borders to trade in products from other countries. These types of studies are widely used around the world. In the last decade, numerous risk analysis studies have assessed the risk of entry of diseases into the EU via different routes.

After conducting these analyses it is essential to disseminate and share the results to all members of relevant sectors. Knowledge transfer allows risk-based decisions to be made, thereby improving the effectiveness of available resources. A veterinary practitioner's ability to respond and prepare will depend on their knowledge, their prior experience with these types of diseases, and their level of alertness for potential signs of ASF. Updating and disseminating information on existing risks and developments in the sector is a duty and a responsibility of all involved. Preventing existing risks facilitates rapid suspicion, early detection, and efficient action in cases of emergency.

KEYS FOR EARLY DETECTION

The period between the entry of the disease into a farm or country and its detection is known as the high-risk period. During this time, the disease spreads easily in the absence of any preventive barriers. This can be facilitated by the legal movement of infected animals prior to suspicion

> Continuing education courses, in addition to drills (either virtual or in the field), are among the best mechanisms by which information can be shared and risks prevented.

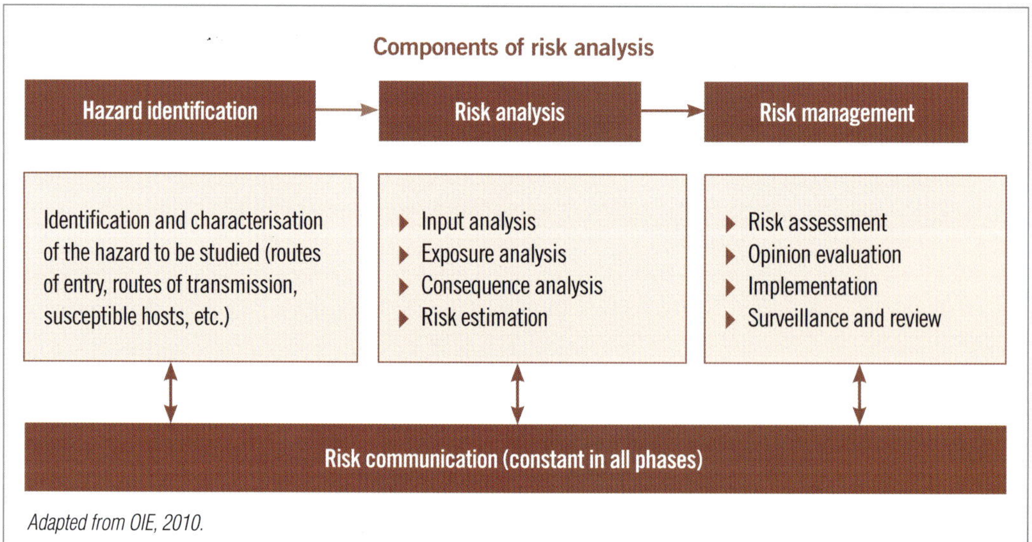

Figure 2. Structure of the risk analysis process of the World Organisation for Animal Health.

of the disease. The longer this period, the greater the risk that the disease spreads to other territories and the greater the potential losses. For the most recent ASF epidemics in the EU, detection time was estimated at 1–3 months. Despite the fact that in Europe the virus was detected relatively late, effective control measures were rapidly implemented, mainly thanks to the high quality of the existing traceability system.

The following are some of the most common reasons for failed early detection of ASF and other exotic diseases:

- The farmer is the first to observe the clinical signs and may subsequently apply a treatment without the knowledge of their veterinary practitioner. Administration of treatments delays disease detection, since it can alter both the clinical signs and the lesions observed.
- The clinical signs are not always obvious or identical to those observed in experimental conditions. In the field, concomitant processes are often present, complicating identification of the disease.
- Private veterinary surgeons are informed late.
- If a private veterinary surgeon decides to collect samples, these can only be sent to private laboratories. These laboratories are not linked to official laboratories and will not be able to diagnose diseases such as ASF, for which high-level biosafety measures are required.
- Finally, it is important to bear in mind that nobody wants to be the first to declare an outbreak of this type of disease.

> In case of doubts regarding notifiable diseases, the best option is to always speak with an official veterinary surgeon.

The following are some actions that can prevent the aforementioned detection failures:

- Establish better communication and greater interaction between farms, private veterinary surgeons, and official veterinary surgeons.
- Create channels to promote communication and collaboration between private and official laboratories.
- Transmit up-to-date risk information to private and official veterinary surgeons on a regular basis.
- Pay greater attention in the field.
- Conduct simulation programmes, provide epidemiological information on risk factors, etc.
- Reduce the official diagnostic time to less than 24 hours to minimise impact on farmers.

With a view to improving early field detection of diseases such as ASF, continuous monitoring systems are being developed using sentinel animals. These systems quantify the most important parameters at the moment of disease, including animal movements (Fig. 3), water consumption, and temperature. Monitoring of movement is achieved using an online night-vision video surveillance camera that tracks pigs continuously for 24 hours, after which the recorded data are analysed using artificial vision algorithms. Decreases in movement compatible with the onset of ASFV infection can be detected before the appearance of fever or other clinical signs, and in some cases before or at the same time as real-time PCR detection of the virus in blood.

This new system represents a significant improvement with respect to those currently used: it is noninvasive, offers greater sensitivity and early detection capacity, and is inexpensive and user-friendly. The development of new technologies and their implementation on farms would help increase the efficiency of early disease detection, as well as reducing the risk of positives between sampling time points.

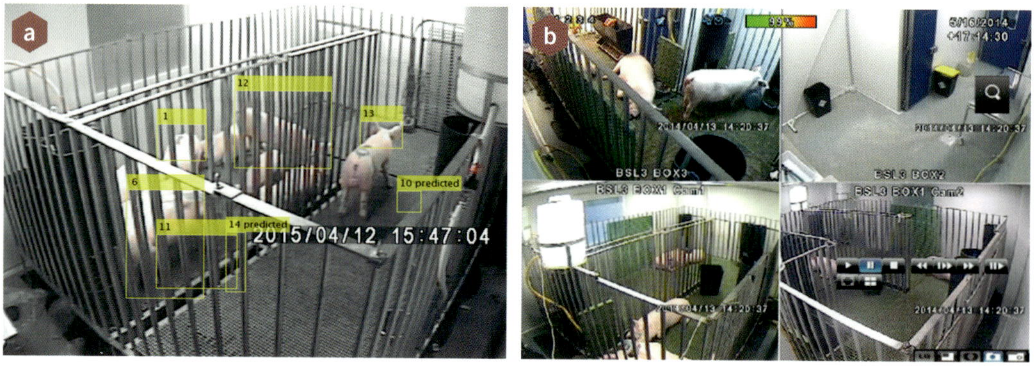

Figure 3. Schematic showing of a new method for the diagnosis of infectious diseases that involve fever through monitoring of changes in movement. Experimental studies were conducted to monitor animals 24 hours a day using online video cameras (Fernández-Carrión et al., 2017).

HOW AND WHEN SHOULD DISEASE BE SUSPECTED?

In cases of notifiable diseases the veterinary practitioner plays a very important role, since they establish the presumptive diagnosis and subsequently communicate their suspicion to the official veterinary services, which are responsible for taking the necessary actions. Establishing suspicion is the most important link in the entire early detection chain. To do this, the clinician must first analyse in detail the specific characteristics of the farm.

Critical data to consider

- The farm's productive and reproductive parameters.
- Movements in recent weeks (entry of animals, material, feed, visitors, etc.).
- Treatments performed in recent days.
- Diseased animals.
- Unusual lesions or clinical signs.
- Abnormalities observed by the farmer and farm workers.
- Notification of any incident that may have violated the farm's biosecurity measures.

Changes in some of these parameters that may be cause for alarm include a large number of deaths in a short period of time, the appearance of fever, and any unusual event that may impact farm biosecurity (e.g. visits, entry of vehicles from outside the farm). In all cases it should be possible to establish a presumptive diagnosis after interviewing the farmer and inspecting the animals. Animals should always be inspected beginning with the area of lowest risk and ending with the area of greatest risk, leaving animals with suspected infection (i.e. those in which the farmer observed the problem) to limit potential spread of the disease to other areas of the farm. Animals with clinical signs and those in close contact with them should be inspected in order to detect any shared pattern of lesions or clinical signs.

Next, necropsies should be performed on the relevant animals, including those that have died in the preceding 24 hours and those that are ill and need to be slaughtered for humane reasons. When performing necropsies extreme biosecurity measures should be implemented to minimise the risk of disease spread. One such measure is the use of insecticides to avoid the presence of flies. Studies have demonstrated

Clinical signs and lesions indicative of potential ASF infection

The variability of the clinical presentation will depend on the virulence of the isolate. The following clinical signs are typically observed:

- Fever (hyperthermia)
- Depression, prostration
- Anorexia
- Hyperaemia, haemorrhagic skin lesions
- Dyspnoea, cough
- Constipation followed by diarrhoea
- Nervous clinical signs (ataxia, paresis)
- Death without apparent clinical signs

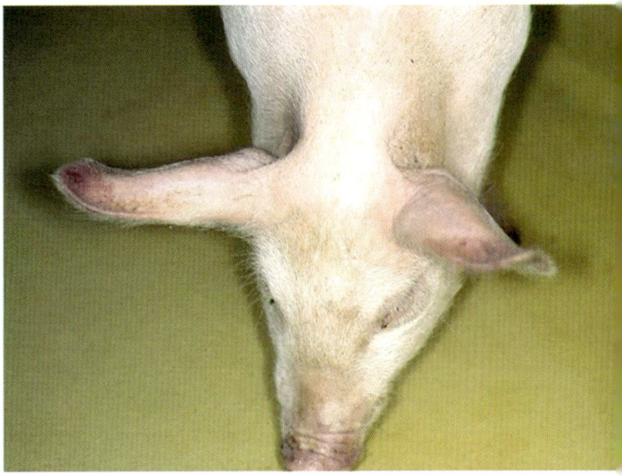

Figure 4. Redness and cyanosis of the ear margins (SUAT-Visavet).

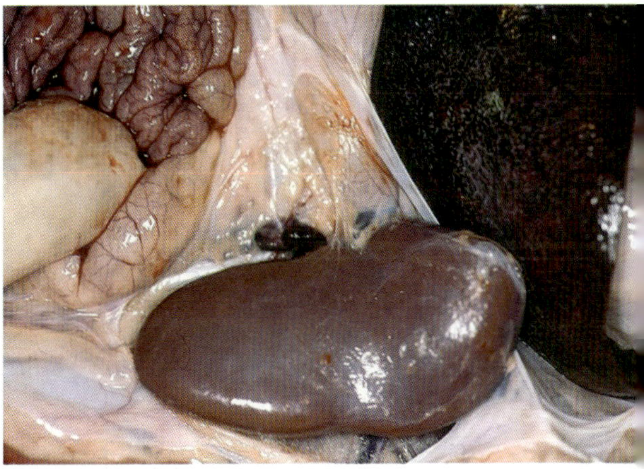

Figure 5. Haemorrhagic renal lymph node (SUAT-Visavet).

that flies can act as vectors by mechanically transmitting or ingesting ASFV. After necropsy, animal remains should be appropriately disposed of or stored in a sealed container. They should never be removed from the farm. The area in which the necropsy was performed should be cleaned and disinfected, and disinsection performed.

Pigs affected by ASF can present with a wide variety of clinical signs and nonpathognomonic macroscopic lesions. In acute cases the most common lesions are erythema and cyanosis of the skin, especially on the ears, snout, distal extremities, and abdomen (Fig. 4); haemorrhagic congestion of the lymph nodes (Fig. 5); splenomegaly (Fig. 6); and spleen lesions (Fig. 7).

Clinical presentations of field and experimental infections can differ. Similarly, the characteristics of a given disease in a previously disease-free area can differ to those in an endemic region. It is therefore essential to consider the possibility that we may encounter other diseases with clinical signs and lesions similar to those of the suspected disease. Most of these diseases are not notifiable and have far less serious consequences. It is especially important to establish a correct differential diagnosis upon encountering a case compatible with ASF.

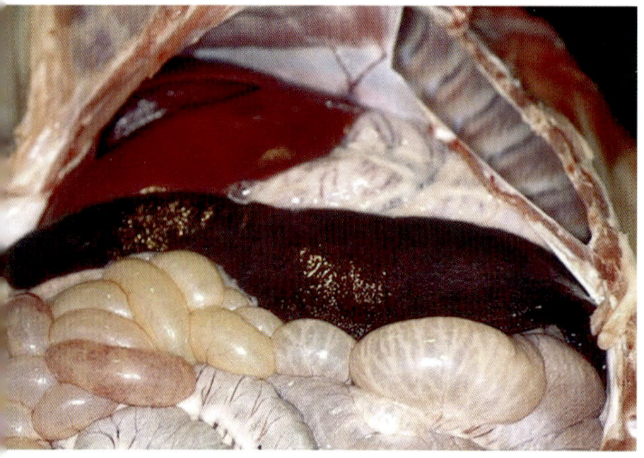

Figure 6. Hypertrophied spleen crossing the abdominal surface and presence of congested intestinal loops (SUAT-Visavet).

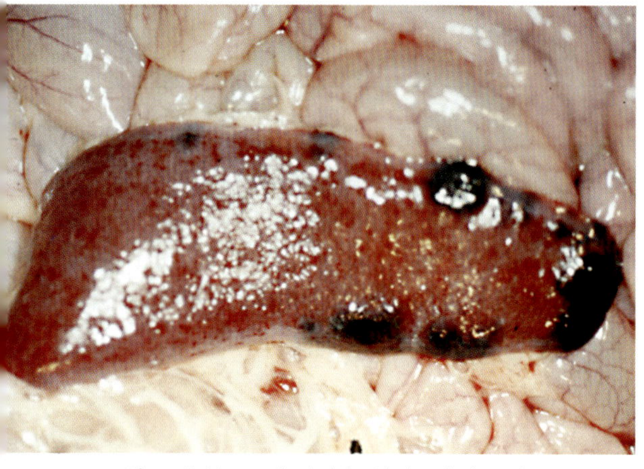

Figure 7. Haemorrhagic infarct lesions in the spleen (SUAT-Visavet).

The following diseases should be included in the differential diagnosis of ASF: classical swine fever, salmonellosis, erysipelas, acute pasteurellosis, viral encephalomyelitis, streptococci, leptospirosis, circoviriosis (porcine dermatitis and nephropathy syndrome, and post-weaning wasting syndrome), and coumarin poisoning.

If ASF is suspected based on the data collected about the farm and the results of the animal inspections and necropsies, this information should be communicated to the official veterinary services as soon as possible.

An official veterinary surgeon must be immediately notified of any clinical or epidemiological suspicion of ASF.

ACTIONS IN CASE OF SUSPECTED ASF INFECTION

Once suspicion of ASF has been communicated, official veterinary surgeons will launch the official disease control protocol, which entails implementation of the control measures described in the contingency plans. These contingency plans are designed according to the administrative structure of each country. However, in all cases the actions to be taken upon suspicion and confirmation of an outbreak or case of ASF should be clearly described in detail. In general, official veterinary surgeons will be tasked with visiting the farm in question to assess the situation. If appropriate, they will report the suspicion and take the appropriate measures to avoid spread of the disease until the focus is confirmed/ruled out.

It will be necessary to conduct a complete census to register and identify all animals and thereby prevent the movement of any animal from the affected farm. Another key element of the response is an epidemiological enquiry, which should be completed by the owner of the animals to try to identify the source of the infection as well as possible contacts with other farms. This can help avoid the appearance of secondary foci.

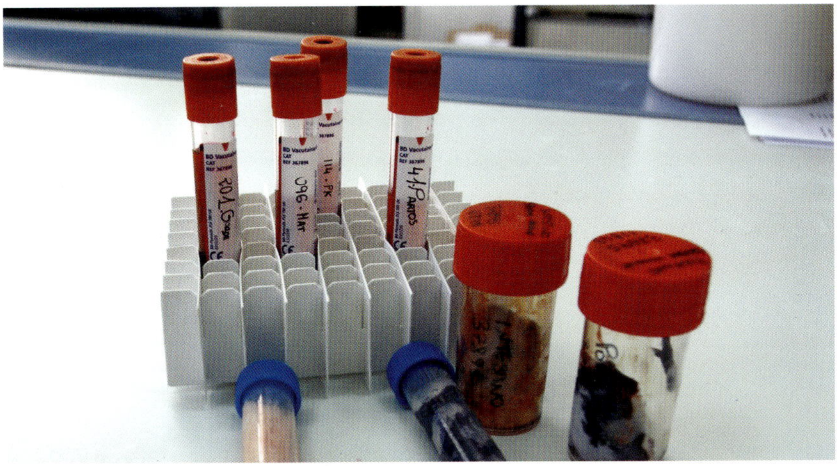

Figure 8. Triple packaging: primary container.

Collection and transport of samples is another key aspect of the protocol. In the case of ASF, care should be taken when preparing samples for transport. In general, this is carried out under the supervision of the official veterinary services of each country. Samples must be triple packed:

- Primary container: sealed, airtight tube in direct contact with the sample (Fig. 8).
- Secondary container: airtight and durable, with absorbent material to collect fluids in case of breakage (Fig. 9).
- External container: protects against damage. Cardboard box or cool box with refrigerant material inside for proper conservation of the samples. The relevant documentation should be attached externally (Fig. 10).

The samples should be shipped to the national reference laboratory after providing prior notification of the situation and the estimated date of arrival.

In cases of suspected outbreak another key measures is to prohibit the entry and exit of any type of animal or product into or out of the farm until the presence of ASF has been confirmed or ruled out. The owner of the farm should be informed of this precautionary measure, and should collaborate to ensure that it is correctly implemented.

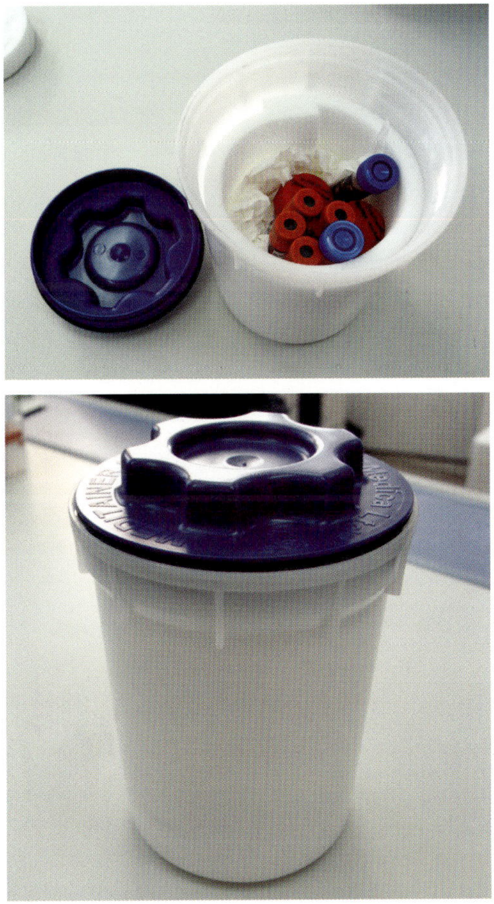

Figure 9. Secondary container containing the primary containers plus absorbent material.

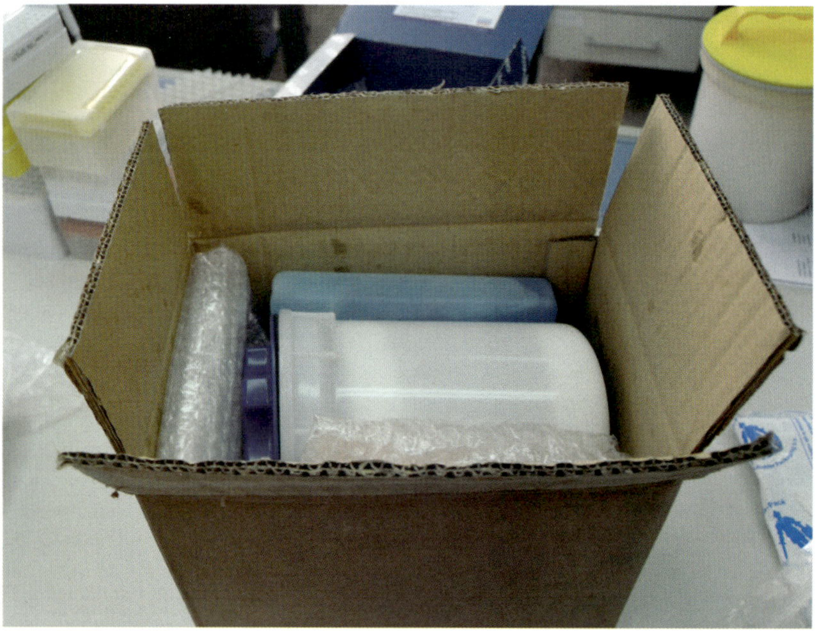

Figure 10. External container (cardboard box containing refrigerant material).

Samples of choice in suspected cases of ASF

- Blood (EDTA) and serum
- Tonsils
- Lymph nodes (gastrohepatic, retropharyngeal, submandibular, and renal)
- Spleen and kidney
- Lung
- Bone marrow (a useful option when sampling from putrefying carcasses)

Protection and surveillance radii of 3 and 10 km, respectively, should be established. Within this protected area measures will be implemented to facilitate detection of new cases, and thereby prevent spread to new areas.

If deemed necessary, these measures will be extended to other farms with which there has been suspected contact. These farms will be identified, to the extent possible, based on the findings of the epidemiological enquiry. The farm will remain in this situation, unable to move animals or products, until suspicion of disease has been confirmed or ruled out based on the laboratory results.

ACTION AND RESOLUTION OF A FOCUS OF ASF

Upon confirmation of an ASF outbreak it is important to have a knowledge of the mandatory control measures, the necessary actions to restore normalcy, and the potential consequences.

WHAT SHOULD BE DONE AFTER CONFIRMATION OF A FOCUS OF ASF?

To confirm an outbreak of ASF for the first time in a given region, positive results must first be confirmed by the national reference laboratory. At the national level, notification of the competent authorities and the World Organisation for Animal Health (OIE) of the presence of the disease is the responsibility of the head of veterinary services, who should provide all necessary information. These types of immediate notifications are published on the OIE website in near real time *(http://www.oie.int/wahis_2/public/wahid.php/Diseaseinformation/Immsummary)*, ensuring transparency and free communication of information. At the farm level, official veterinary surgeons will immediately launch a protocol that will include mandatory slaughter of the animals present on the farm.

Animal slaughter

Animals must be slaughtered as soon as possible, always adhering to current animal welfare regulations. The carcasses of slaughtered animals must be appropriately destroyed in accordance with local legislation.

The presence of a notifiable disease requires slaughter of all susceptible animals (infected and uninfected) present on the affected farm.

Detailed epidemiological enquiry

The goal of the detailed epidemiological enquiry is to gather all relevant information to elucidate the origin of the disease and to locate possible secondary outbreaks and anticipate possible infections on other farms. In addition to the information obtained from the farm census, as well as information on farm management and the clinical course of the disease, the enquiry gathers data on the entry and exit of people, products, animals, and vehicles during the 60-day period prior to detection of the focus. Farms that have had direct contact with the affected farm in the preceding 2 months should be considered suspicious, and surveillance measures implemented.

Cleaning and disinfection

Cleaning and disinfection will be carried out throughout the operation by an entity certified by the competent body, under the supervision of an official veterinary surgeon.

All material present should be removed, and the area thoroughly cleaned with water and detergents that eliminate any remaining organic matter. In areas in which there may be traces of grease it can be useful to use a degreasing agent prior to disinfection. Next, all surfaces and materials are disinfected using appropriate concentrations of the recommended products. The products should be left in place for 24 hours on all surfaces to be disinfected. A final round of cleaning and disinfection is performed after 7 days.

Detergents can be added to disinfectant solutions (15 ml per 5 litres of disinfectant) to increase their disinfectant power.

Tracing and destruction of products and materials

Based on an estimated date of potential entry of the virus into the farm, we can retrospectively trace the outflow of animals, as well as the movement of any products capable of transmitting the disease (e.g. meat, slurry, manure, bedding).

All material should be treated using procedures that ensure destruction or inactivation of the virus.

This tracing procedure should also be simultaneously applied to the control and surveillance zones around the affected farm (radii of 3 and 10 km, respectively).

> The objective of creating these zones is to prevent and control the spread of the disease. The control and surveillance zones are areas with radii of 3 and 10 km, respectively, around the disease focus.

Within these areas the movement of products and animals susceptible to the disease is frozen, and any farms within are visited to ensure the absence of disease.

Each time a new outbreak is identified corresponding protection and surveillance zones are created. These zones can potentially overlap with those of other foci. Actions continue in the control areas until the absence of disease is confirmed based on the results of clinical and serological analyses. Control measures must be implemented for a minimum period of time. Serology is a very useful tool to rapidly and effectively determine the extent of an infection. It is usually applied in areas adjacent to the declared focus to determine whether the infection has spread. It is a simple and inexpensive method that enables analysis of many samples in a short period of time.

> Cleaning and disinfection of the areas in which animals are slaughtered and necropsied, and of all utensils used, should be performed before and immediately after slaughter/necropsy. The remaining facilities should be cleaned in the days immediately after.

Evaluation of the health and ecological status of wildlife

The role of wildlife in ASF outbreaks is an important factor that should always be borne in mind, particularly in outbreaks on extensive farms. Wild boar are susceptible to ASF, are capable of transmitting the virus and the infection to domestic pigs, and can even act as a source of infection. Conversely, the virus can be transmitted from domestic pigs to wild boar, which subsequently act as a reservoir of the virus.

In response to notification of ASF in wild boar, pigs in the affected area must be kept in enclosures to prevent contact with wildlife. A surveillance system is established for domestic pigs, as well as a series of control measures to be applied to wild boar.

A surveillance programme should be implemented to ensure the rapid and safe removal of carcasses, which are the most likely to present some form of disease. Analyses should also be performed on a proportion of animals killed during hunting or population control programmes (Fig. 1).

Evaluation of the presence of vectors in the area

Another element that should be studied before beginning repopulation of the farm is the presence of vectors capable of maintaining and transmitting ASFV. Ticks of the genus *Ornithodoros* spp. *(O. moubata* in Africa and *O. erraticus* [Fig. 2] in the Iberian Peninsula) have been identified as vectors and reservoirs of the virus. These soft ticks can survive for long periods of time and remain infective with ASFV for years (Fig. 3).

This type of tick tends to stay on the animal for only a few minutes, and prefers to remain underground in dark and humid areas, typically in old stone structures with many wall cracks in which it can hide. Given this behaviour, it is extremely important to confirm the presence or absence of this vector on affected farms (Fig. 4).

This is ideally achieved using CO_2 traps in which ticks can be captured for subsequent analysis (Fig. 5).

In addition, serological tests can identify animals that have been bitten by this tick species

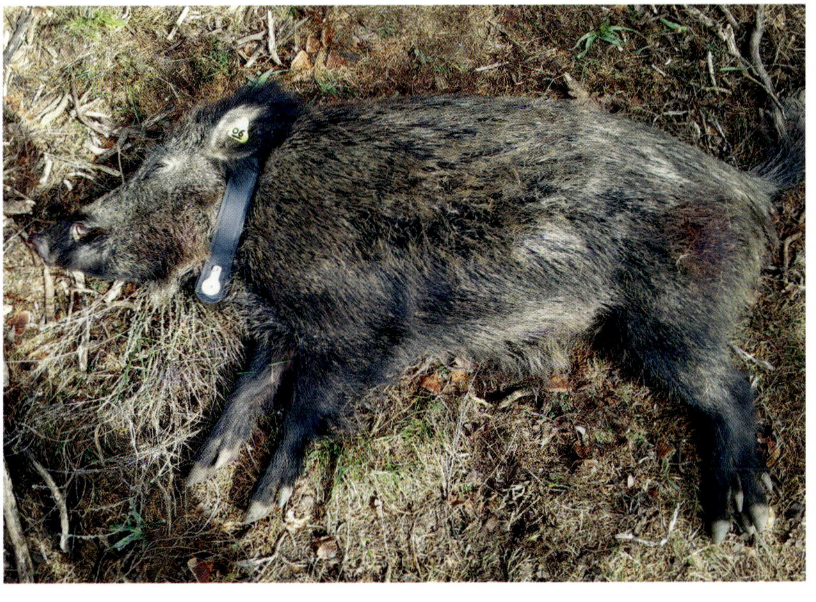

Figure 1. Wild boar captured for sampling and implantation of a geolocation device to monitor its movement.

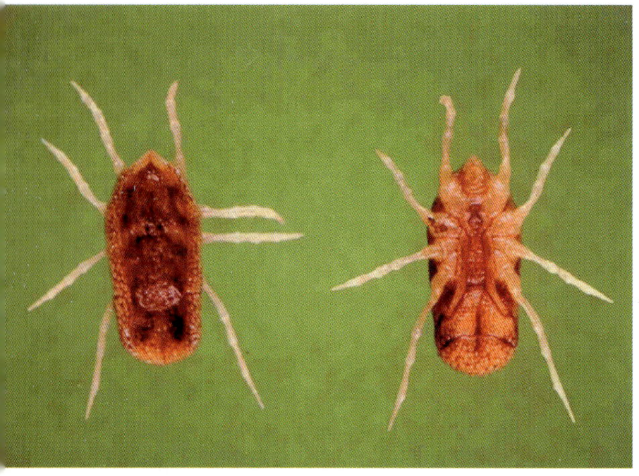

Figure 2. *Ornithodoros erraticus.*

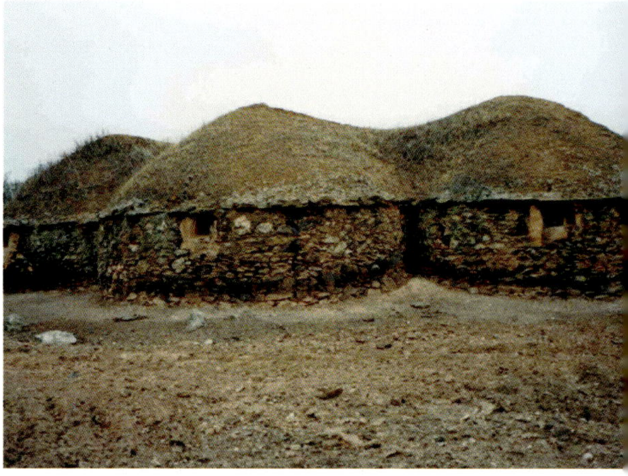

Figure 3. Pigsty in which *Ornithodoros erraticus* is commonly found.

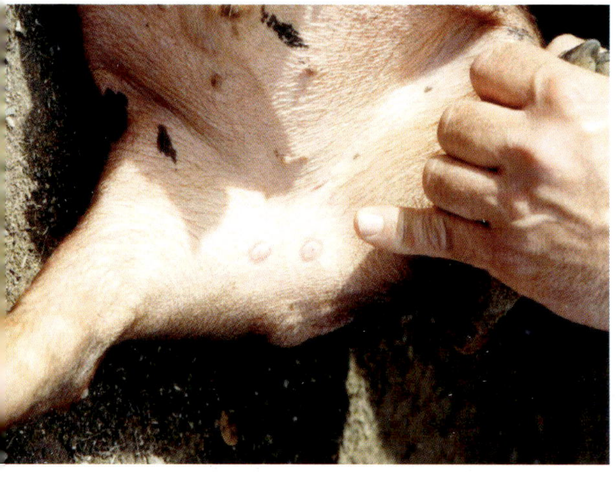

Figure 4. Tick bites on the belly of a pig.

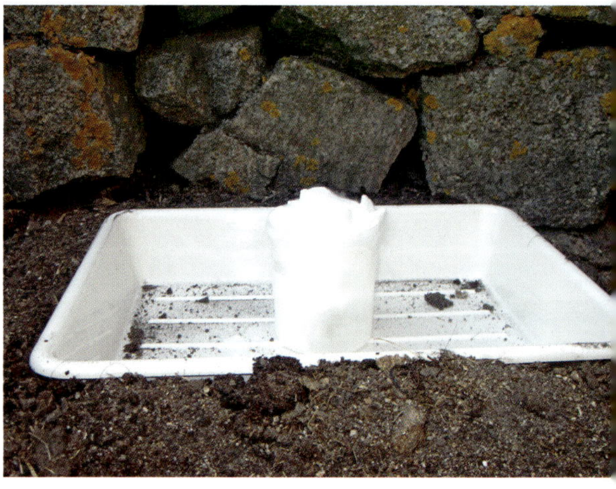

Figure 5. CO_2 traps made with dry ice to capture *Ornithodoros erraticus* on a farm.

by detecting antibodies against the salivary glands of the tick. This serological test allows identification of farms on which ticks are present. Disinsection of the facilities should be performed if the result is positive, although this can be very challenging. However, multiple serological studies and direct searches for ticks conducted in affected areas, including Sardinia and Germany, have failed to reveal the presence of these ticks. Similarly, the results of direct searches conducted in Eastern Europe were negative.

If tick involvement in a focus of ASF is suspected, this period can be extended to up to 6 years.

Use of sentinel animals

Finally, complete repopulation of an affected farm should ideally be preceded with the introduction of sentinel animals. Farms should never be repopulated within less than 40 days after completion of the final cleaning and disinfection operations.

Repopulation is carried out by introducing ASF-free animals from areas free of restrictions associated with the disease focus. Animals must be housed in the previously affected farm and should undergo periodic serological tests. Until the results of these tests are negative none of the newly introduced animals can leave the farm. Serological tests should be performed 45 days after introduction of the animals. It should be noted that the aforementioned periods are standard recommendations, and can vary depending on the biosecurity measures of the farm and the status of neighbouring farms. After this period the farm can proceed with complete repopulation and restoration of normalcy, provided that the sentinel animals test negative for ASF.

CONSEQUENCES OF A FOCUS OF ASF

The entry of this disease always has very negative consequences for both the affected farm and the country in which it is located. As seen with ASF outbreaks in Europe and Asia, the true scope of the disease's impact can be difficult to quantify.

One way to quantify losses or costs associated with a disease outbreak is to separate direct from indirect costs.

Direct costs

- Visible costs: these include the cost of dead animals and those incurred controlling the outbreak (slaughter and destruction of infected animals, cleaning and disinfection, etc.).

Indirect costs

- Impact on human health: fortunately, ASF is not zoonotic and therefore has a limited public health impact.
- Indirect control costs: includes the costs of surveillance, additional personnel, etc.
- Income lost: market closures, price decreases, loss of consumer confidence, and other possible negative economic effects on the sector.

The economic and political consequences of diseases such as ASF tend to be more severe than the health impact. They include both the direct costs incurred due to the outbreak and other associated costs (closure of markets, decreases in product prices, surveillance costs, etc.). Sometimes variations in the price of products can lead to changes in market trends, giving rise to illegal trade.

This is a major problem in ASF-free countries, where piglet prices are high. In countries such as Poland and Romania outbreaks of ASF and consequent market closures have led to decreases in piglet prices. This price difference can foment illegal importation of piglets, with consequent health risks.

As with human diseases, it is very difficult to calculate the costs associated with any animal disease, as this involves several sectors and numerous parameters, many of which are difficult to quantify.

BIBLIOGRAPHY

1. Acevedo P et al., 2006. Factors affecting wild boar abundance across an environmental gradient in Spain. *Acta Theriologica*. 51(3):327–336.
2. Alexandersen S et al., 2002. Quantities of infectious virus and viral ARN recovered from sheep and cattle experimentally infected with foot-and-mouth disease virus O UK 2001. *J Gen Virol.* 83(8):1915–1923.
3. Arias M et al., 2017. Gaps in African swine fever: analysis and priorities. *Transbound Emerg Dis.* 65: 235–247.
4. Boadella M et al., 2011. Six recommendations for improving monitoring of diseases shared with wildlife: examples regarding mycobacterial infections in Spain. *Eur. J. Wildl. Res.* 57(4):697–706.
5. Cottam EM et al., 2008. Transmission pathways of foot-and-mouth disease virus in the United Kingdom in 2007. *PLoS Pathog.* 18(4):e1000050.
6. Chmitelin I., Moutou F, 2002. Foot and mouth disease: lessons to be learned from the experience of France. *Rev Sci Tech.* 21(3):731–737.
7. Fernández-Carrión E et al., 2017. Motion-based vídeo monitoring for early detection of livestock diseases: The case of African swine fever. *PLoS One.* 12(9):e0183793.
8. Food and Agriculture Organization of the United Nations (FAO), 2019. *ASF Situation Update.* Available at: www.fao.org/ag/againfo/programmes/en/empres/ASF/Situation_update.html (last date accessed: 22 January 2019).
9. Grupo SUAT-VISAVET, 2018. *Simulacros digitales de enfermedades animales.* Available at: www.sanidadanimal.info/sanidadanimal/es/cursos/simulacros.html
10. International Civil Aviation Organization (ICAO), 2005. *Technical instructions for the safe transport of dangerous goods by air. Guidance document for Infectious substances.* Available at: www.wfcc.info/new/Documents/icaoAddendum.pdf (last date accessed: 14 October 2019).
11. International Federation for Animal Health, 2012. *The Costs of Animal Diseases.* Available at: https://healthforanimals.org/component/attachments/attachments.html?task=attachment&id=34 (last date accessed: 14 October 2019).
12. Jurado C et al., 2017. Why is African swine fever still present in Sardinia? *Transbound Emerg Dis.* 65:557–566.
13. Jurado C et al., 2018. Relevant measures to prevent the spread of African swine fever in the European Union domestic pig sector. *Front Vet Sci.* 5:77.
14. Keuling O et al., 2013. Mortality rates of wild boar *Sus scrofa* L. in central Europe. *European Journal of Wildlife Research*, 59(6):805–814.
15. Laevens H et al., 1998. An experimental infection with classical swine fever virus in weaner pigs. I. Transmission of the virus, course of the disease, and antibody response. *Vet Q.* 20(2):41–45.

16. Laevens H et al., 1999. Experimental infection of slaughter pigs with classical swine fever virus: transmission of the virus, course of the disease and antibody response. *Vet Rec.* 145(9):243–248.
17. Leme RA, Alfieri AF, Alfieri AA, 2017. Update on Senecavirus infection in pigs. *Viruses.* 9(7): E170.
18. León EA, 2012. Foot-and-mouth disease in pigs: current epidemiological situation and control methods. *Transbound Emerg Dis.* 59 (Suppl 1):36–49.
19. Li L et al., 2019. Infection of African swine fever in wild boar, China, 2018. *Transbound Emerg Dis.* 66(3):1395–139.
20. Martínez-Avilés M et al., 2017. Early Detection of Infection in Pigs through an Online Monitoring System. *Transbound Emerg Dis.* 64(2):364–373.
21. Martínez-López B et al., 2008. Quantitative risk assessment of foot-and-mouth disease introduction into Spain via importation of live animals. *Prev Vet Med.* 86(1-2):43–56.
22. Martínez-López B., Pérez A.M., Sánchez-Vizcaíno J.M. 2009. A stochastic model to quantify the risk of introduction of classical swine fever virus through import of domestic and wild boars. *Epidemiol Infect.* 137(10):1505–1515.
23. Mur L et al., 2017. Serological surveillance and direct field searching reaffirm the absence of *Ornithodoros erraticus* ticks role in African swine fever cycle in Sardinia. *Transbound Emerg Dis.* 64(4):1322–1328
24. Mur L et al., 2012a. General framework for the risk assessment of African swine fever introduction into the European Union. *9th International Congress of Veterinary Virology.* Madrid, Spain. 4–7 September, 2012.
25. Mur L, Martínez-López B, Sánchez-Vizcaíno JM, 2012b. Risk of African swine fever introduction into the European Union through transport-associated routes: returning trucks and waste from international ships and planes. *BMC Vet Res.* 8:149.
26. Mur L et al., 2017. Serological surveillance and direct field searching reaffirm the absence of *Ornithodoros erraticus* ticks role in African swine fever cycle in Sardinia. *Transbound Emerg Dis.* 64(4):1322–1328.
27. Oleaga A, Pérez Sánchez R, Encinas Grandes A, 1990. Distribution and biology of *Ornithodoros erraticus* in parts of Spain affected by African swine fever. *Veterinary Record,* 126(2):32–37.
28. Oleaga A, Pérez Sánchez R, Encinas Grandes A, 1990. Distribution and biology of *Ornithodoros erraticus* in parts of Spain affected by African swine fever. *Veterinary Record,* 126(2): 32–37.
29. Pérez-Sanchez et al., 1994. Relationship between the persistence of African swine fever and the distribution of *Ornithodoros erraticus* in the province of Salamanca, Spain. *Veterinary record,* 135(9); 207–209.

30. Sánchez-Vizcaíno JM, Arias M, 2012. African swine fever. In: Zimmerman J, Karriker L, Ramirez A, Schwartz K, Stevenson G (eds): *Diseases of Swine*, 10th ed. Blackwell Publishing Professional, Ames, Iowa, pp. 396–404.
31. Sánchez-Vizcaíno JM et al., 2015. An update on the epidemiology and Pathology of African swine fever. *Journal of Comparative Pathology*. 152:9–21.
32. Sánchez-Vizcaíno JM, Mur L, Martínez-López B, 2013. African swine fever (ASF): five years around Europe. *Vet Microbiol.* 165(1-2):45–50.
33. Sánchez-Vizcaíno JM et al., 2015. An update on the epidemiology and pathology of African swine fever. *J Comp Pathol.* 152(1): 9–21.
34. Spanish Ministry of Agriculture and fisheries, food and environment (MAPAMA), 2019. *Manual práctico de las operaciones en la lucha contra la peste porcina africana.* Available at: www.mapa.gob.es/es/ganaderia/temas/sanidad-animal-higiene-ganadera/manualpracticoppa572019_tcm30-428107.pdf (last date accessed: 16 October 2019).
35. Spanish Ministry of Agriculture, Fisheries and Food, Dirección general de sanidad de la producción agraria, *Spain–Classical swine fever 1997–13th report.* Madrid, Spain.
36. Standing Veterinary Committee. 1997a. *Information on classical swine fever in Germany.* Bundes Ministerium für Landwirtschaft, Germany.
37. Standing Veterinary Committee. 1997b. *Classical swine fever 1997 – 13th report.* Spanish Ministry of Agriculture, Fisheries and Food, Dirección general de sanidad de la producción agraria, Madrid, Spain.
38. Suli T et al., 2017. Body temperature and motion: Evaluation of an *online* monitoring system in pigs challenged with Porcine Reproductive & Respiratory Syndrome Virus. *Res Vet Sci.* 114:482–488.
39. Terpstra C, Dekker A, Wensvoort G, 1992. Classical swine fever and swine vesicular disease: familiar diseases back in the Netherlands. *Annual report of the Institute for Animals Science and Health* (CDI-DLO), Lelystad, Netherlands. pp. 23–29 (Dutch).
40. Thompson D et al., 2002. Economic costs of the foot and mouth disease outbreak in the United Kingdom in 2001. *Rev Sci Tech.* 21(3): 675–687.
41. Vanthemsche P, 1996. Classical swine fever 1993–1994 Belgium. *Pig J.* 37(1): 43-53.
42. Williams DR, Matthews D, 1988. Outbreaks of classical swine fever in Great Britain in 1986. *Vet Rec.* 122(20):479–48.
43. World Organisation for Animal Health (OIE), 2019. *Wahis database.* Available at: www.oie.int/es/sanidad-animal-en-el-mundo/portal-wahis-datos-de-salud-animal/ (last date accessed: 22 January 2019).
44. World Organisation for Animal Health (OIE), 2010. *Handbook on Import Risk Analysis for Animals and Animal Products.* World Organization for Animal Health, Paris, France.